Fifty Ways To Leave Your Blubber

Fifty Ways To Leave Your Blubber

Vince Lambri

Illustrations by Louis Krefsky

ISBN-13: 9781523899029
ISBN-10: 1523899026
Library of Congress Control Number: 2016904205
CreateSpace Independent Publishing Platform
North Charleston, South Carolina

Introduction

have written *Fifty Ways to Leave Your Blubber* to help anyone with weight loss, fitness, exercise, and nutrition. It is my hope that these simple, commonsense guidelines will allow people to be healthy and happy as well as enjoy their lives to the fullest.

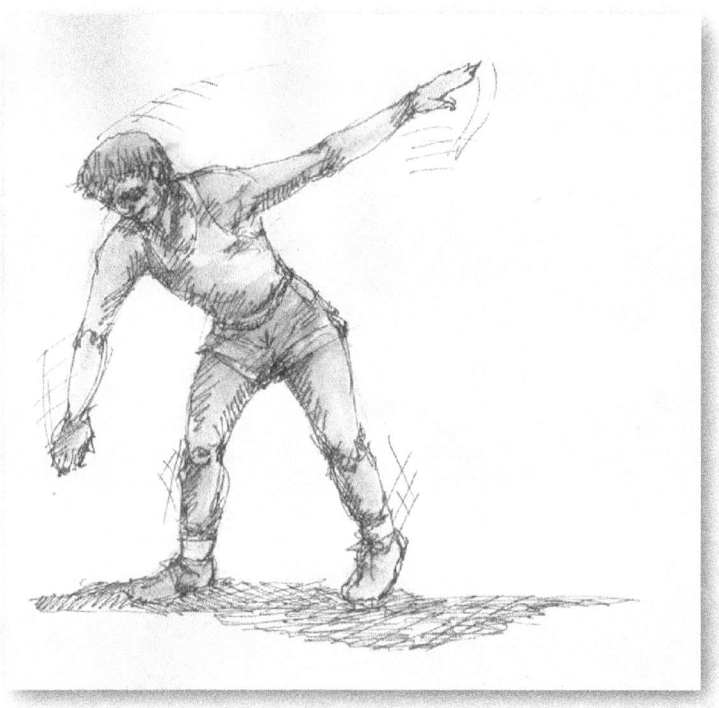

Table of Contents

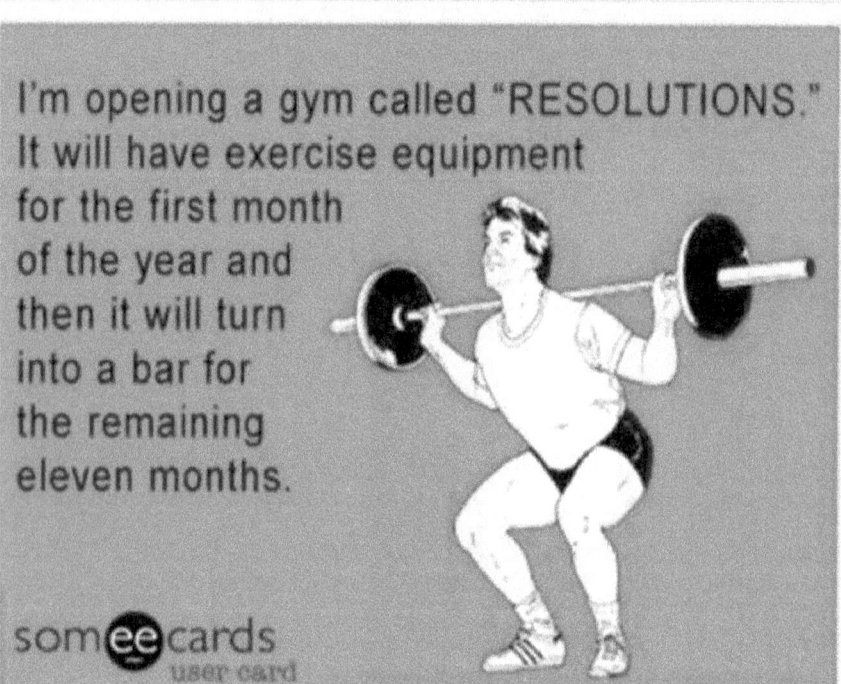

Appetizers

Get Started on the New You

1

A Perfect Ten

Ten Ways to a Healthier Life

1. Exercise regularly to increase your energy level
Regular cardiovascular and strength-training exercises reduce body fat and improve lean muscle. This results in a real increase in metabolism, greater levels of energy, and reduced stress.

2. Use proper exercise form and techniques for the best results
Performing an exercise correctly allows you to efficiently firm and strengthen your muscles. You will avoid injury and see results faster.

3. You've got to move it to lose it—aerobic activity is a must
Regular cardiovascular or aerobic activity burns calories, which leads to fat loss. Aerobic activity is also necessary to strengthen the most important muscle in your body—your heart.

4. Excessive amounts of calories, not fat, will lead to weight gain
Eating too many calories, not fat, each day leads to unwanted weight gain. Eliminating fat from you diet will not necessarily lead to weight loss. A moderate amount of fat is essential for proper health. It gives us a feeling of fullness when we eat, preventing us from overeating.

5. Eat often to eat light

Eating five to six meals per day promotes weight control and increased metabolism. Skipping meals causes you become too hungry, which leads to overeating when you do eat. Your body can't use all the food at one time, so it will store the excess as fat. Skipping meals also slows down your metabolism and makes you feel lethargic.

6. Take vitamins and supplements

Vitamins and supplements augment your body's ability to change and achieve your fitness goals, whether your goal is body fat loss, toning and definition, or lean muscle-mass gains. They also provide essential nutrients that you can't get from food, especially when you are on a caloric-restricted diet in order to lose body fat weight.

7. Strength train with resistance tubes, exercise machines, or free weights

All types of exercise are beneficial. Your choice depends on your location, fitness level, and lifestyle. Exercise machines provide stability and support but are expensive and usually found at gyms or health clubs. Free weights can be used at both health clubs and at home. They require knowledge of proper exercise technique to avoid injury. Resistance tubes are inexpensive, are safe for all fitness levels, and can be used anywhere.

8. Variety is key in sustaining your workouts and maximizing your results

You should vary your workouts in order to achieve your best results and avoid boredom. Change the type of exercises you do, the equipment you use, the number of sets or repetitions you perform, the amount of weight you lift, and the days you work out. Depending on your fitness level, you should change your routines every two to six weeks. Individuals who have exercised longer and are in better shape need to change more often than someone who has just begun to exercise.

9. Perform the correct amount of sets and repetitions

You should do between one to four sets of an exercise, depending on the time you have to work out and the number of different muscle groups you are exercising. You should try to do between six to fifteen repetitions properly per set. If you can't do six repetitions, then the weight is too heavy; if you can do fifteen repetitions easily, then the weight is too light.

10. *Fifty Ways to Leave Your Blubber* can work for you

Fifty Ways to Leave You Blubber can help you achieve the benefits of a healthy lifestyle. Its practical and commonsense fitness, nutritional, and lifestyle tips provide beneficial guidance in all aspects of health and fitness to everybody.

2

Start Me Up

Warm Up for Resistance Training

t is very important to properly warm up prior to your resistance training workouts. Proper pre-workout warm-ups increase circulation to your muscles. This allows for greater muscle usage, increased lifting efficiency, and, most importantly, injury prevention. Below are some useful tips to help you with your warm-ups.

Do At Least Five Minutes Of Light Aerobic Activity

Always do at least five minutes of low-intensity aerobic activity prior to your workouts. Some good suggestions are treadmill walking or stationary bicycle riding. Do not overdo it so that you are too tired to work out hard. Also, you can do additional five-minute aerobic intervals between exercises to keep your metabolism up for greater caloric expenditure.

Stretch, But Don't Overstretch

Gently stretch your muscles to limber up and improve circulation. Do not overstretch to achieve greater flexibility or range of motion. Prolonged stretching for flexibility improvement should be done after your resistance exercises.

Do One Light Set First

Try to do one light set before adding additional weight or increasing resistance. Practice your form, checking for proper alignment, posture, range of motion, repetition speed, abdominal support, and breathing.

Avoid Prolonged Rest Intervals

Try not to rest for too long between sets or exercises. Your body will cool down, and you will lose the benefits of your warm-up. Keep your rest intervals between forty-five seconds and three minutes, depending on the amount of resistance you are using.

Stay Focused On Your Workouts

Do not stray from your exercise program, daydream, or socialize too much while you are working out. Stay focused and complete your workout with minimal interruptions. You can relax after you are finished.

3

Stay Regular

Keep Your Weekly Workouts Consistent

The key to long-term health, getting in good shape, maintaining your fitness levels, and obtaining the best results is to stay regular with your workout schedule. Consistent workouts will optimize your exercises and make it possible to achieve your goals.

Frequently, people start out exercising too much—sometimes every day. Eventually, they may become tired or disillusioned with the lack of results. You should start exercising no more than two or three times per week and stick to that schedule. Occasionally, if you feel up to it, you can add an additional workout or two, but always maintain your two to three weekly workouts. Below are some helpful suggestions to keep you regular.

Schedule Your Workouts

If you have a busy or hectic schedule, it is a good idea to schedule your workouts as if they are doctor's appointments. You should pick times that are convenient and avoid excuses that cause you to change your schedule.

Stay Realistic

Keep your workout time realistic. A two- to three-hour workout five to six times per week is something that very few people can do for an extended period of time. Do only what is possible. Remember that this is a lifetime commitment.

Reward Yourself For Each Workout

Reward yourself for sticking with your workout schedule. Go out and buy something for yourself or participate in leisure activities with family and friends.

Pay A Penalty For Missed Workouts

Fine yourself ten dollars every time you miss a scheduled workout. You can take this penalty money and use it to buy your reward when you adhere to your schedule.

Don't Work Out Too Much To Make Up For Lost Time

If you miss a workout, do not double up on the next workout to make up for lost time. It simply won't work, and you may injure yourself. This is a bad habit that will eventually lead to poor results.

Have A Backup Plan

Make sure there is enough flexibility in your schedule to allow for a new workout time in case you miss a workout. This will reduce stress and make exercise seem less like it is just another chore.

4

The Skinny on Body Fat

Body Fat Basics

Body fat percentages, along with circumference measurements, are more indicative methods to determine weight loss and fitness conditioning than total body weight. Most people wish to tone up, lose weight, gain muscle, or reshape their physiques. This often involves not only body fat loss but also an increase in lean muscle mass. Stepping on a scale will not tell you if your weight loss is mostly body fat. Also, lean muscle gains often cause an increase in total body weight. Therefore, it is better to measure body fat percentages to assess whether fitness or health goals are being attained.

Body fat percentage is simply the percentage of fat your body contains. Women have a higher body fat percentage than men because men proportionally have more muscle tissue, therefore lowering body fat percentages.

The following scale describes body fat percent ranges and categories. Keep in mind that as we age, our body fat percentage increases at an average rate of 1 percent per year after the age of twenty-one. The average age in the table below is thirty-five years. If you are younger, you should be on the lower end of the category range. If you are older, you will be at the upper end of the category range.[1]

---

1 The information in this table is taken from the American Council on Exercise.

Classification	Women—Body Fat %	Men—Body Fat %
Essential Fat	**10–12%**	**2–4%**

This is the essential fat necessary for basic health and survival. Individuals in this category or lower are undernourished and may have an eating disorder or a medical condition.

Athletes	**14–20%**	**6–13%**

Individuals in this category include many professional athletes, people who exercise intensely, and individuals with genetically low body fat percentages.

Fitness	**21–24%**	**14–17%**

This is the range that most people should strive for as a goal. Most individuals can achieve these measurements with proper, regular exercise and dietary habits.

Acceptable	**25–31%**	**18–25%**

This category includes most adults who do not exercise regularly. It also includes individuals who have genetically high body fat percentages but exercise and diet properly.

Obese	**32% plus**	**25% plus**

These individuals are genetically predisposed to higher body fat or are sedentary and do not exercise or eat properly. This category has the highest risk of medical complications associated with high body fat. Fortunately, this group can make the largest reductions in body fat and gain the greatest health improvements.

5

Supplemental Reading

Guidelines for Taking Vitamins and Supplements

There is much debate today concerning the pros and cons of taking nutritional supplements. While most supplements can be beneficial, the wrong supplement or improper dosage can cause serious and even fatal results.

The main reason you should take supplements is to augment your diet with essential nutrients that may not be available in sufficient quantities from your daily food intake. This is especially true for people on calorically restrictive diets necessary for weight loss. Other common reasons are performance enhancement, muscle gain, and antiaging regimens.

If you are currently taking nutritional supplements or are considering taking supplements, below are some helpful guidelines to follow.

Get A Medical Exam
Before taking any supplements, get a checkup from your physician. You may have a physical condition that a particular supplement may contraindicate. Discuss your supplement plan with your physician and follow any recommendations.

Ask Fitness Professionals
Physicians are usually well versed in medical knowledge but don't always know the latest research on supplements. Ask your pharmacist, personal trainer, nutritionist, or health-food-store salesperson for additional information.

Learn About The Supplements On Your Own

Do not rely on the advice or word of others as your only source for information on supplements. Do some research on your own to find additional information. The Internet is a good place to start.

Avoid Strange Brews, Concoctions, Or Potions

Use supplements from a name-brand company that provides pharmaceutical-grade products and lists all the ingredients. Avoid unusual or unknown items.

Follow The Dosage

Make sure to follow the recommended dosage for a particular supplement. This is true for the dosage amount, ingestion timing, and water and food intake.

More Is Not Better

Do not assume that ingesting a greater amount of a particular supplement will increase its effects. It won't. Over dosage is the main reason why people become sick, injured, or suffer even worse consequences.

Discontinue Using Supplements If You Experience Side Effects

Even though you may be medically and physically fit enough to take a particular supplement, if you feel any unusual side effects, stop at once. Your body is trying to tell you that this supplement may not be right for you.

6

See You at the Club

Guidelines for Health Club Selection

C hoosing the right health club may often determine your success in achieving your fitness goals. There are several important factors that should be considered when selecting a gym or health club.

Location
Your health club should be conveniently located near your home or workplace. If it is difficult to get to or involves an excessive amount of traveling time, eventually you will stop using its services.

Condition Of The Equipment
Check the condition of the equipment. While most health clubs provide a wide variety of exercise machines, poorly maintained equipment may indicate a gym with financial problems. You may be more likely to injure yourself with exercise equipment that has been neglected.

Number Of People In The Health Club Or Gym
When you are given a tour of a gym or health club, check to see if it is overcrowded. If there are too many people in the gym waiting for machines or cardio equipment, you may want to consider a different place where you will not waste your time.

Amenities

Amenities such as child care, weight loss and nutritional counseling, spa services, and a juice bar can make a prospective health club more attractive and suitable for your needs.

Cleanliness

A clean health club is usually indicative of a well-maintained and financially secure facility. Check the locker rooms and bathrooms before deciding to join.

Staff

Find out if the personal trainers and nutritional counselors are properly certified. Make sure that they are capable of providing the professional assistance you need.

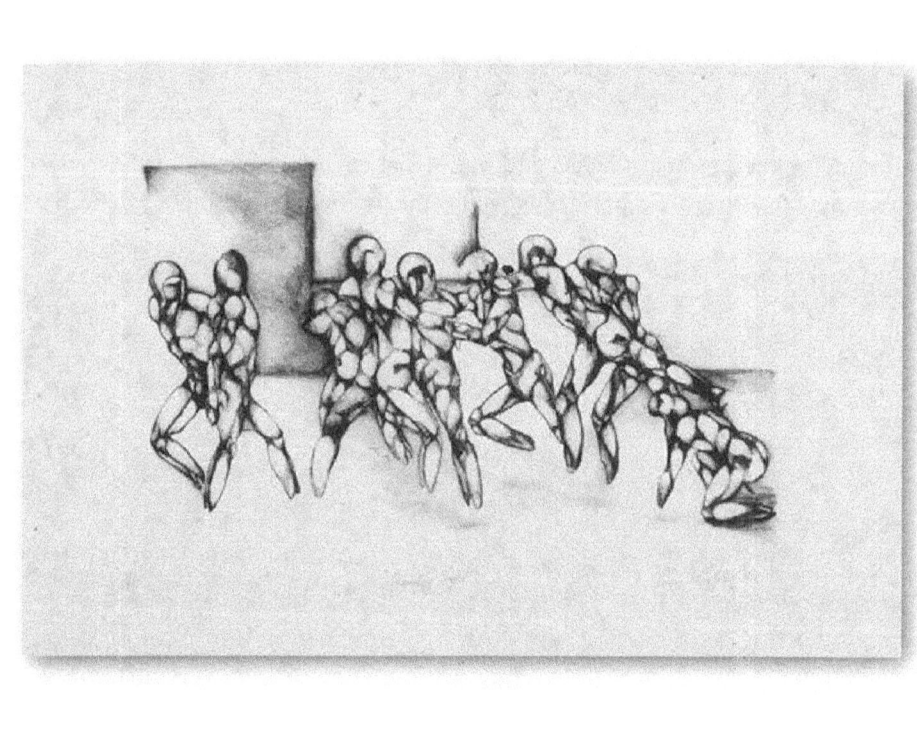

First Course

Better Nutrition and Eating

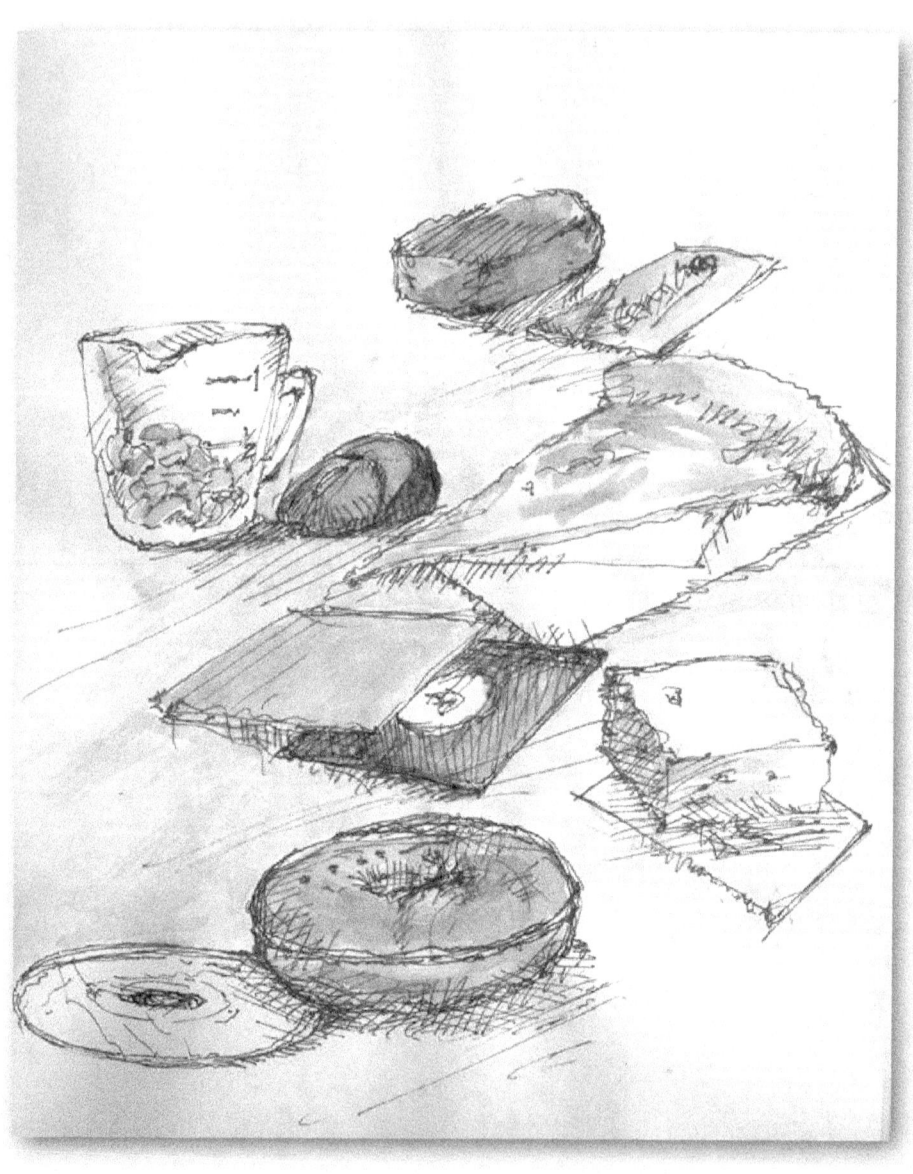

7

Size Does Matter

Be Aware of Portion Size When Watching Your Weight

Many people who are watching their weight are somewhat knowledgeable about which foods are healthy and what to eat. Unfortunately, without an awareness of portion size, people can still consume too many calories, even though they feel that they are eating healthily. This is especially true of individuals who eat out often, as restaurant portions tend to be much larger than recommended serving sizes.

Below are some examples of portion sizes:

- A one-ounce slice of American cheese (105 calories) is about the same size as a computer disc.
- Three ounces of cooked lean meat (240 calories) is about the size of a credit card half an inch thick.
- Half a cup of cooked pasta (400 calories) is about the size of a computer mouse (two and a half inches by one and a quarter inches).
- A four-ounce plain bagel (310 calories) is about the size of a CD-ROM.
- A regular slice of cheese pizza (225 calories) should fit inside a standard business envelope.
- A two-inch standard square brownie (125 calories) is about half the size of a business card.

8

Eat Often and Weigh Less

Healthy Food Consumption

To improve your body, look and feel better, and improve your overall health, you should get in the habit of feeding your body more often. Numerous studies conducted by leading nutrition and diet experts have concluded that when an individual eats more often, metabolism is accelerated, resulting in more calories burned. When you consume five to six small, nutritious meals per day, the food is more efficiently absorbed than a typical eating pattern of one to three large meals per day.

Excess food that is consumed with large meals will be stored as body fat. When an individual eats only one to three meals daily, his or her body's homeostatic mechanisms interpret the long periods between meals as a possible starvation scenario. This leads to a greater tendency to store the excess food as body fat in order to compensate for these long periods of perceived fasting.

When you eat every few hours, you will feel like you have more energy. You will also avoid spikes in insulin levels. This may reduce your appetite and food cravings. Above all, you will create a metabolic environment that supports fat loss and muscle gain, which will transform your body in the shortest amount of time.

9

Leave a Bite and Lose the Pounds:

A Simple Method to Lose Weight

Today the media is full of conflicting advice regarding weight loss. The American Medical Association recommends one type of diet, while Dr. Atkins recommends another. Everyone seems to have the answer to permanent weight loss along with tests results to justify their claims.

I feel that since people come in all shapes, sizes, ages, and fitness levels, the results an individual will obtain from a particular diet regimen will vary. Additionally, genetics play an important part in overall weight loss.

While we wait for the government as well as the science and medical communities to finally figure out the best diet, I offer the following simple tip to help you lose pounds and keep unwanted weight from coming back.

Try to leave one bite of food at each meal. Although this may not seem like much, it can add up to a reduced consumption of one hundred to two hundred calories daily. This can lead to a loss of over one pound per month, or over twelve pounds in one year.

10

Don't Jump In

Timing Exercise and Meals

Many people say that timing is everything. This is especially true for exercise workouts and eating meals. Proper timing of workouts and meals can enhance performance and results while avoiding undesirable consequences.

After a person eats a meal, the body diverts blood to the internal organs of the digestive system in order to process the food that has just been eaten. When a person participates in a vigorous exercise workout, the body diverts blood to the working muscles involved in a specific activity. If exercise is performed too soon after eating, your body will prematurely take away blood from your digestive system. This often results in abdominal cramps and nausea.

There are several guidelines to keep in mind when timing your workouts and meals. Usually, you can do a light to moderate workout after waiting one hour after a meal. For strenuous or long-duration workouts, it is best to wait three hours after food consumption. You should not skip meals or exercise if you feel hungry. To maintain optimal workout performance, avoid intense exercise if you have not eaten for more than four hours. A light snack or energy bar can be consumed before any type of workout, especially if you feel hungry or have not eaten in over four hours.

11

Veggies

Nutrition Tips for Vegetarians

Many people and celebrities, such as Paul McCartney, Bill Clinton, and Carrie Underwood, are choosing to become vegetarians in one form or another. Below are several nutritional tips for vegetarians.

Avoid Eating Too Many Carbohydrates
Vegetarians may often increase the amount of carbohydrates they eat as a percentage of their total caloric intake. Avoid overconsumption of pasta, bread, and desserts.

Use Soy Protein To Increase Dietary Protein
Total protein intake can be a problem for vegetarians. Use soy products or soy food substitutes as an alternative source of protein. Most supermarkets now carry soy-based items, such as veggie burgers and smart hot dogs.

Increase Fruits And Vegetables In Your Diet
Increasing fruits and vegetables in your diet will reduce insulin spikes as well as reduce cravings for sweets.

Snack On Nuts

Nuts are a good source of protein and taste good. Also, if you have to remove their shells, as in the case of pistachio nuts, you'll eat more slowly and avoid excessive consumption.

Drink Protein Shakes

Protein shakes are an excellent source of supplemental protein for both vegetarians and non-vegetarians. They also facilitate a healthy habit of eating five to six times per day.

Ask Restaurants For Vegetarian Entrees

More restaurants now provide vegetarian entrees. These are often not on the menu, so ask for them. Also, when making reservations, ask for vegetarian meals. They can be prepared ahead of time, thus avoiding excessive waiting.

Make Sure To Consume Essential Fat

Not all fats are bad for you like trans fats are. There are good fats known as high-density lipoproteins (HDLs), omega-3s, omega-6s, and healthy essential fatty acids, such as linoleic and linolenic acids. Olive oil, nuts, safflower oil, and coconut oil are good sources of these nutrients. Vegetarians and non-vegetarians should include these foods in their diets. They are important for skin and cell-membrane health and actually promote body fat metabolism. They can also reduce appetite, overeating, and food cravings.

12

The Numbers Game

Don't Be a Slave to the Scale

Weight loss and weight management are common goals for many people. It is often useful and desirable to measure weight to evaluate progress, modify diet plans, and change exercise programs. However, people may become obsessive in weighing themselves. This could be counterproductive and ultimately lead to a regain of weight that has been lost.

A person's weight varies by as much as five pounds throughout the day. This fluctuation usually results from varying amounts of water uptake and food ingestion. Medications, illness, activity levels, menstrual cycles, and hormonal changes can also affect total body weight.

If a person who is actively trying to lose weight weighed him or herself repeatedly throughout the day, that person would invariably see random weight gains and losses that are inconsistent with his or her weight management efforts. This could be frustrating and depressing. These fluctuations, which have nothing to do with body fat loss, will also skew daily comparative scale readings.

It is recommended that you weigh yourself no more than once per week and at the same time of the day. The readings will more accurately reflect actual weight loss. Body fat measurements are also more indicative of total body fat loss than a simple weight measurement on a scale. Finally, place more emphasis on other forms of measurement and feedback, such as the way your clothes fit, to evaluate the success of your weight-loss efforts.

Entrees

Exercise and Fitness

WHO ARE THESE CHARACTERS?

WORKOUT GIRL

13

Stay Active, Stay Calm

Aerobic Exercise and Hypertension

Regular aerobic exercise is considered essential by many physicians for short-term and long-term control of hypertension. Aerobic exercise appears to reduce both systolic and diastolic blood pressures, cardiac output, and peripheral arterial resistance. Below are some helpful tips to keep in mind when working out.

Consult With Your Physician
If you are diagnosed with hypertension, consult with your physician before beginning any form of exercise. Ask for specific exercise guidelines and how your hypertensive medication could affect your workouts.

Extend Warm-Up And Cooldown Times
Extend your warm-up and cooldown times to approximately ten minutes. Gradually build up to your maximum exercise intensity and then slowly reduce your intensity. This will avoid excessive blood pressure increases as a result of your exercise.

Exercise Five To Six Times Per Week
For optimal control of your hypertension from exercise, it is recommended that you exercise five to six times per week and anywhere from twenty to sixty minutes at a time.

Incorporate Interval Training

Try to incorporate some form of light interval training into your activities. This will make your aerobic activities more efficient and less monotonous.

Avoid Excessive Impact

Since it is recommended that an individual with clinically diagnosed hypertension exercise five to six times per week, it is a good idea to incorporate aerobic activities that have little or no impact, such as swimming or using elliptical machines. This will help avoid joint and muscular discomfort.

Keep Intensity Low To Moderate

Keep your exercise intensity low to moderate. This will also avoid higher heart rates and blood pressure. Initial exercise intensities should be 40 to 65 percent of your maximum heart rate. Over time, the intensity may be increased to 55 to 70 percent.

14

Spot Reduction Does Not Hit the Spot

A Common Exercise Mistake

M any people have a particular area on their body that they wish to improve in appearance. They think they can achieve this by reducing body fat in a specific location. Too often they "over exercise" this area in an attempt to target body fat loss.

For instance, it is common for women to want a reduction in the size of their hips and thighs. They participate in exercise routines that emphasize the muscles in these areas. If you go to a health club, you'll usually see many women spending a great deal of time on the hip adductor and abductor machines in an attempt to reduce hip and thigh body fat. While their motivation and commitment are commendable, their efforts will not bring them the results they desire.

Typically, men try to firm up their abdominal area to achieve six-pack abs. They will spend an inordinate amount of time doing hundreds of sit-ups and other abdominal exercises in a vain endeavor to flatten their midsections.

These approaches to specific body fat reduction will not lead to targeted decreases in body fat. Over exercising a specific area may lead to both intra- and intercellular muscle enlargement in the very spots a person is trying to reduce.

With regard to exercise, in order to improve your appearance, work out your entire body with a combination of proper weight-training exercises and a variety of regular aerobic activities. This will lead to an improvement in overall muscle tissue and an increase in metabolism. The resulting additional caloric expenditure will cause increased body fat utilization and a reduction in total body fat.

Unfortunately, where this body fat comes off is determined genetically. You simply cannot burn it off at a particular spot. However, if you stick to a regular exercise routine and a healthy lifestyle, your body fat will eventually decrease in the desired locations. Above all, you will gain the many health benefits of total body conditioning.

15

A Change Will Do You Good

Modify Your Resistance Training Workouts

Everyone who exercises regularly, regardless of individual goals, will, at times, become stagnant or bored with the same workout routine. This usually leads to a lack of improvement or a plateau in conditioning. It is therefore important to modify your workouts to keep you challenged and motivated as well as to continue with increased results. Below are some suggestions that will help.

Change The Type Of Resistance
Use different types of resistances to increase muscle-fiber recruitment. For instance, if you primarily use free weights, try to use tubes, machines, cable exercises, or manual resistance.

Change Your Resistance Progressions
Change the way you increase or reduce weight during a set. If you have been increasing weight after each set, try starting out heavy and then decreasing. You could also keep the weight the same.

Change Your Exercises

For a period of time, do different exercises for a particular body part. Avoid doing the same exercises over and over. Performing the same exercises will limit your results and may lead to muscle imbalances and injuries.

Change The Order Of Your Exercises

If you usually work specific muscle groups one at a time, try to do a few routines that involve circuit training. You can repeat the circuit two to four times.

Mix Aerobic Activity In Between Sets

Try to mix short aerobic activities in between exercises or circuits. For example, you could jog for five minutes in between your back and shoulder exercises. If you do five to six exercises, you will incorporate about thirty minutes of aerobics into your routine.

Incorporate All Your Workout Tools

Use all these tools to do different workouts. One day, you could use tubes; the next day, you could use free weights. You could even do a set with tubes and then the next set with free weights. The more you change, the better your results.

16

Home on the Range

Range of Motion—Know Your Limits

The term "range of motion" is often used to describe the degree of a person's joint movement and flexibility. Sometimes individuals and trainers are confused about the precise understanding of proper range of motion.

According to the National Academy of Sports Medicine, there are three range-of-motion types, each with its own specific definition.

Passive Range Of Motion

This range of motion can be defined as the one achieved when an outside force causes movement around a joint. This external force can be your own body, muscles from another part of your body, another person, external weight, or a machine. It is usually the maximum range of motion a joint can move.

Active Range Of Motion

This is the range of motion that can be achieved through the action of the agonist muscles for a specific joint movement. For example, the active range of motion for elbow flexion is the movement of the forearm by the action of the biceps. It is typically less range than the passive range of motion.

Resisted Range Of Motion

This can best be defined as the range of movement a person can move with resistance and remain in control of that movement. It varies with resistance and will decrease as resistance increases.

People should limit their resisted range of motion when doing exercises with heavy weights. This applies to beginners and advanced individuals. Heavy weights moved through maximum passive range of motion can cause strain and injury to joints, ligaments, and weaker stabilizer muscles. When people are participating in strength-training exercises, passive and full active ranges of motion are not necessary to gain results.

17

A Stable Situation

Improved Stability Brings Improved Results

Strong stabilizer muscles are essential for maximizing your fitness results. Too often, individuals concentrate on exercising the major muscle groups while neglecting stability training. Weak stabilizers will prevent people from lifting heavy weights, even though their major muscles can handle it. Below are some useful tips to keep in mind.

Always Use Proper Form

Proper form will maximize results while, at the same time, minimizing injury. By concentrating on proper exercise form, you will strengthen your stabilizer muscles. Work out with a personal trainer to learn correct exercise form and alignment.

Vary Your Workouts

Changing your workout routines will employ different muscles. You will also use the same muscles in slightly different ways. This variation will utilize and train the stabilizer muscles effectively.

Use Tubes

Exercise or resistance tubes employ elastic resistance. This type of resistance, along with the unstable nature of tubes, will strengthen the stabilizers. Resistance tubes also allow for more varied types of movement during an exercise.

Limit Your Range Of Motion

Do not exceed your resisted range of motion and avoid unnecessary body movements. Always maintain correct posture and alignment.

Go Slowly

Always do each repetition slowly. This allows you to concentrate on proper form. The old adage that fast movements burn fat and promote muscle tone is nonsense.

Perform Stabilizer Muscle Exercises

When exercising, incorporate specific exercises to train your stabilizer muscles. Rotator cuff exercises are extremely beneficial and easy to do.

18

Expedite the Situation

Reduce Workout Time with Active Rest

Very often, you may feel that you have no time to exercise. You may perceive your workouts to be a long, time-consuming task. Also, if you have exercised for a long period of time, you may become unmotivated to continue with your regular workouts.

One way to reduce the length of your workouts, increase motivation, and save time without reducing results is to employ the techniques of active rest when exercising. Essentially, active rest refers to training methods where a different exercise is performed between sets of a particular exercise. This is done instead of passively resting between each set.

For instance, you can alternate antagonistic muscle groups, such as switching between bicep curls and triceps extensions. Other useful antagonistic muscle pairings are latissimus dorsi pull downs with shoulder presses, chest presses with back rows, leg adduction with leg abduction, and leg extensions with leg curls.

Another active rest technique is to alternate aerobic activity between sets or exercises. For example, you could walk or jog on a treadmill for one to two minutes between sets or three to five minutes between different exercises.

This routine will also keep your muscles warmed up as well as increase metabolism and caloric expenditure during workouts.

By following these simple variations, you may find that your workouts will be more stimulating and challenging. You'll also save time, which will make it easier to incorporate regular workouts into your weekly schedule.

19

True Grip

Proper Handgrip Techniques for Strength Training

Sometimes it is the little things in life that have a significant effect on the big picture. When it comes to resistance strength training, a proper handgrip is an important factor in achieving successful results.

It is a common tendency to tightly grip weights, handles, weight bars, or exercise machines. This may lead to muscle cramps, hand discomfort, and, most significantly, a reduction in the amount of weight you will move or lift.

If you were to tightly scrunch up your toes on your feet, you would find it difficult and almost painful to walk. The tension in your toes and feet greatly reduces the coordination and strength of your leg muscles. Even though walking is a simple physical action, you may find it difficult to sustain. Your toes and feet will begin to ache after a short period of time.

This situation is analogous to gripping tightly with your hands. The additional strain leads to fatigue of the forearm muscles, resulting in reduced performance. This is especially true for exercises such as the latissimus dorsi pull down, back row, and bicep curl. Your forearms and hands ache before you fully exhaust the larger muscles, forcing you to back off or stop your set prematurely.

You should make a conscious effort to keep your handgrip as light as possible. If possible, try to use a slightly open grip or utilize the assistance of a spotter or personal trainer. Try to not flex your wrists, and keep your hands and forearms aligned straight.

20

Sudden Impact

Tips for Reducing Impact Discomfort and Injury

Discomfort and injury from excessive impact motions can adversely affect your exercise workouts, particularly your aerobic activities. Constant trauma to your lower limbs can cause foot, knee, and hip-joint problems. Sometimes the discomfort can be severe enough that you may have to stop exercising and seek medical treatment. Below are some useful tips that will help you reduce impact injuries.

Start Out Slowly

Begin an exercise workout by warming up. If you are just starting to exercise regularly, do not try to do too much at first. Gradually build up your running speed and distance.

Incorporate Variety

Whether you have been running and exercising for a long time or are just starting out, it is best to incorporate different types of aerobic activity. Do not jog or run as your only method of exercise. Alternate your workouts by using a cross trainer or StairMaster or by taking a spinning class.

Run Lightly

When you are running, jogging, or walking, try to "run lightly." Imagine you are running over a bed of hot coals. While you will not reduce the actual force of your impact, by picking your legs up faster, you reduce the shear forces on your joints that are caused by forward momentum.

Use Proper Running Shoes

Make sure you have good running or walking shoes. Ensure that they fit properly, provide adequate cushion and ample support, and are not worn. You may want to see a podiatrist and get a pair of orthotic inserts made specifically for exercise.

Rest

If you experience discomfort or pain after jogging or running, rest a day or two to let it subside. Do not try to work through the pain. If it persists, see your physician. Problems treated early often resolve themselves faster than a chronic problem that is ignored.

21

Variety is Spicy

Change Up Your Aerobic Workouts

The many health benefits of cardiovascular exercise are well known. Regular aerobic activity improves heart and respiratory function, increases metabolism, reduces blood pressure, relieves mental stress, and is essential to weight loss and weight maintenance.

When it comes to cardiovascular activity, changing and adding variety to your workouts will increase the results that are gained. If an individual performs the same activity, his or her body will physiologically adapt to that particular type of exercise. The body will then become more efficient and require less energy to do that same workout. This will result in a decrease in overall desired health and fitness improvements. Repeating the same exercise in the same way can also lead to injury, boredom, and loss of motivation.

You should try to do at least two to three different types of aerobic activity each week. If you jog or walk a lot, try using a cross trainer, StairMaster, elliptical machine, or a row machine or try swimming. You could take a group fitness class or try a spinning class. If you take the same group fitness class or use the same exercise videotape, try a different one. You can also try to do interval training, whereby you change the speed or intensity during your workout instead of constantly moving at the same pace. Other options include randomly changing the length of your workouts or exercising at different times of the day. Finally, you could substitute your workouts with recreational activities, such as tennis, hiking, cycling, golf, or swimming. Enjoy yourself. You've earned it!

22

Too Tired to Workout

Tips for Exercising When You Feel Tired

At times, everyone feels too tired to work out. There is a general feeling of exhaustion and reluctance to exercise. You just do not feel like making the trip to the gym, lifting, or participating in aerobic activity. For many, this can lead to feelings of guilt, anxiety, and a sense that they are failing to keep in shape.

There are several reasons why you may feel too tired to work out. Understanding them may help you cope or modify your workouts to avoid this malaise.

The first thing you should consider is your level of conditioning and how long you have been exercising regularly. If you have just started exercising and are somewhat out of shape, it is natural for your body to feel exhausted as it tries to adjust to new exercise routines. Also, people who just start out often overdo it in the first few weeks. Some simple solutions would be to rest, avoid working out every day, and avoid workouts of more than an hour.

If you have been working out for a long time and are in fairly good shape, you should take a break for a few days or a week. Your level of conditioning will not be that greatly affected, and you may avoid exercise burnout. When you resume your workouts, you may get more out of them and move off the plateau that you may be stuck on.

Other factors to be considered are the time of day you exercise, the repetitive nature of your workouts, and your current health. If your workday is long and you are faced with a long commute home, it may be difficult to feel energized to work out in the evening. You may want to consider morning or lunchtime workouts as an alternative. If you have been doing the same routine over and over, change your exercises. Go to the gym and use machines that you have never used before or take a new aerobics class. Chronic exhaustion may also be a sign of illness or allergies. Get a checkup from your doctor to see if you are well or need medication.

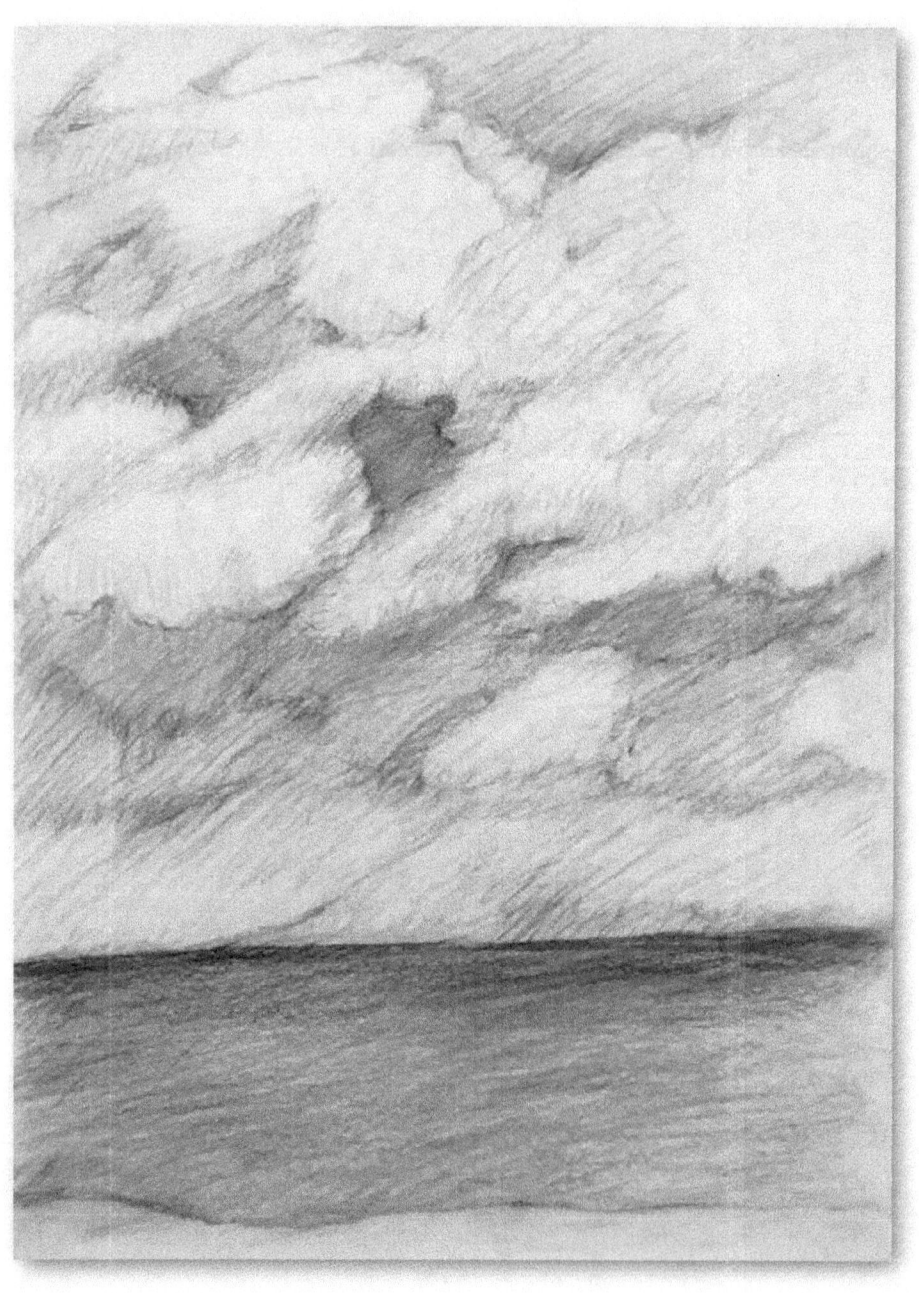

23

Beat the Heat

Smart Tips for Hot-Weather Exercise

During the late spring, summer, and early fall, with temperatures soaring into the nineties and hundreds, exercise can be hazardous and not beneficial unless some commonsense precautions are taken. Below are several safety tips that can help you beat the heat and stay healthy.

Stay Hydrated—Drink Plenty Of Fluids

Proper fluid maintenance is critical when exercising in hot weather. An individual should drink at least eight ounces of water before exercise, between five to ten ounces of water every fifteen minutes during exercise, and finally, at least eight to sixteen ounces of water after exercise. An individual, after exercise, may drink low-carb sport drinks to help replenish lost electrolytes. Avoid caffeine or alcoholic drinks.

Time Your Workouts

If possible, schedule your workouts during the morning or evening hours when it is cooler. Avoid intense midday exercise sessions.

Protect Your Body

Wear as little clothing as possible to promote sweat evaporation. Wear light-colored, loose-fitting clothing. Avoid rubberized or 100 percent cotton materials. Use sunscreen with a sun protection factor (SPF) greater than fifteen.

Take It Easy

Don't overwork yourself. Reduce your workout time, preferably by at least 50 percent. Rest every ten to fifteen minutes and avoid exercising outdoors for more than ninety minutes.

Find A Climate-Controlled Environment

Seek out a facility, gym, health club, room, or environment that is air conditioned. Even short periods of time in a cool environment will lessen the risk of heat injury.

Use The Buddy System

If you exercise outdoors, it is a good idea to work out with a friend, neighbor, relative, or coworker. Each of you can check the other for signs of heat exhaustion or heatstroke. It is best to use a personal trainer to monitor your condition during your workouts.

Be Aware Of Signs And Symptoms Of Heat Exhaustion And Heatstroke

Too much activity, sports participation, or exercise can result in heat exhaustion or heatstroke. Overweight individuals, the elderly, children, and people who exercise or participate frequently in sports activities are especially susceptible. Some common symptoms include excessive sweating, muscle cramps, shortness of breath, flushed or reddish skin complexion, dizziness, and fainting.

24

It's Cold as Ice

Running in Cold Weather

R unning, jogging, or walking in cold weather requires some commonsense preparations and precautions. Hypothermia, frostbite, and dehydration are some of the conditions that can occur if you don't protect yourself. Below are practical tips if you venture out in the cold.

Dress To Protect

Make sure you dress warmly. Check the temperature outside so you know how much clothing to put on. Wear your clothing in layers for maximum effectiveness. If possible, wear material close to your body that absorbs perspiration. Avoid removing outer layers as you warm up.

Keep Hands And Feet Warm

Keep your extremities warm. Make sure to wear gloves, warm socks, and running shoes. Also cover your head to prevent excessive heat loss.

Use Sunscreen

Apply sunscreen during the day even though it is winter. The sun's rays will reflect off of snow, intensifying ultraviolet radiation exposure. Also, wear sunglasses or goggles to reduce glare.

Use Proper Footwear And Watch Out For Ice

Make sure your shoes are not worn so that they can provide good traction on slippery or uneven surfaces.

Watch Out For Cars

If you run along the side of a road, be aware of oncoming traffic and other vehicles. Icy roads and high winds may cause erratic driving.

Drink Water; Avoid Caffeine

Make sure you drink plenty of water before, during, and after you exercise to prevent dehydration. Even though it is cold outside, you will lose moisture through perspiration. Avoid caffeinated drinks like hot coffee.

Don't Go Far

Even if you are careful or are in good physical condition, it is a good idea not to go too far or to take an isolated route. Often, cell-phone reception is not very good. If something should happen and you are on a well-traveled road, you can get assistance more easily.

25

Final Ab Solution

New Tips for Flatter Abs

There is much written on the best training techniques for obtaining flatter-looking abdominal muscles and a slim waist. Unfortunately, the truth is that except for a few people, most individuals rarely achieve this goal. Often, this is due to incorrect training, lost exercise opportunities, or boredom from doing too many crunches. Here are some new tips to improve your chances to get flatter abs.

Tighten Your Abs When Doing All Exercises

Whenever you do any exercise—whether it is a shoulder press, leg squat, latissimus pull down, biceps curl, or whatever—make sure to tightly contract your abs during the entire exercise set. This will both train your abs to stay tense and provide greater support for your spine.

Hold Ab Crunches And Avoid Excessive Repetitions

When doing abdominal exercises, like a crunch, hold the contracted position for at least five seconds. By employing this technique, you should be able to do no more than ten to twenty repetitions per set.

Use A Stability Ball To Extend Range Of Motion

Use a stability ball to extend the range of motion of an ab crunch. It allows your upper body to move below the plane of your hips. This will allow for a more efficient movement and better results.

Use A Balance Or Wobble Board

A wobble or balance board will utilize your abdominal muscles to provide both balance and spinal support. This will isometrically contract your abs, which will lead to increased firmness.

Emphasize Back Rows To Improve Posture

An upright postural alignment will make your abdominals look flatter. If you have well-developed abs and low body fat but maintain a slouched stance, you'll still look like you have a paunchy midsection.

Maintain Regular Aerobic Activity

In order to achieve flatter-looking abs and a slender waist, it is necessary to do regular aerobic exercises and activities. This will help burn calories and, along with proper resistance training, reduce body fat.

26

Back It Up

Strengthen the Lower Back

Work- and sports-related back injuries are common problems for both conditioned and unconditioned individuals. It is estimated that 70 to 90 percent of the population suffers some type of lower-back pain or injury. Below are some helpful tips to improve lower-back strength and reduce the probability of discomfort.

Proper Examination And Assessment

If you have had a history of lower-back pain, you should be examined by a physician and assessed by a personal trainer. Determining the cause of your discomfort and areas of weakness is invaluable for proper exercise selection.

Core Strengthening

Strengthening your core will reduce the risk of lower-back pain and injury. All major muscle groups and stabilizers should be exercised in all planes of motion.

Balance Training

Improving your balance will reduce lower-back strain. A wobble board and yoga exercises are particularly effective.

Abdominal Training

Strengthen all your abdominal muscles in order to provide proper support for your lower back.

Posture Improvement

Exercises that improve posture, such as a back row, will enhance vertebral alignment, leading to a reduced incidence of lower-back pain.

Single-Leg Exercises

Engaging in single-leg exercises, such as a squat, will improve balance as well as strengthen hip, hamstring, abdominal, and back muscles.

Use A Stability Ball

Use a stability ball to enhance abdominal range of motion, assist in one-legged exercises, and stretch the lower back. A ball will also provide instability during an exercise, which will lead to increased adaptive muscle stability.

Stretch

Stretch your back, hips, hamstrings, glutes, and neck muscles.

27

Bringing up the Rear

Maximizing Your Glutes

The gluteus maximus is one of the most prominent muscles in the human body. Besides providing a wide array of essential functions, it is also considered an important measure of appearance and fitness. The desire to "firm up the butt" is a common goal. Below are some helpful tips to improve your glutei workouts.

Improve Core Strength

Use a stability ball to improve overall core strength. Any type of exercise can be done on a ball, such as abdominal crunches, bicep curls, triceps extensions, and lateral raises. The demand placed on your glutei to provide stabilization will enhance muscle-fiber recruitment.

Stretch And Improve Flexibility

Tight muscles, such as iliopsoas, hamstrings, hip flexors, erector spinae, adductor magnus, and the IT band, can reduce glutei function. This will result in decreased muscle action and muscle weakness.

Use Balance-Training Exercises

Employ balance-improvement exercises, such as single-leg squats or use of a wobble board. This will also increase glutei function and efficiency, which will lead to faster results.

Do Lunges Or Step-Ups In Different Directions

Do lunges and step-ups in different directions to exercise the glutei in all planes and ranges of motion. Again, this will increase muscle efficiency and strength, ultimately leading to better results.

Straight-Leg Kickback With Tubes

Use a resistance tube loop and place both feet within it. Hold onto a stationary object and kick one leg back as far as you can while trying to keep it as straight as possible. Think of a figure skater that kicks her leg back before making a jump. Hold and return without touching the ground. Repeat with the other leg.

28

The Agony of the Feet

Improper Footwear Can Lead to Pain without Gain

Painful, sore feet can be very uncomfortable and may prevent individuals from exercising properly. Sometimes people ignore foot discomfort and attempt work out through it, ultimately causing substantial injury. This may lead to costly medical treatment and prolonged interruptions in exercise.

Most individuals have a small natural misalignment of their feet. There may be a slight inversion, eversion, pronation, or supination of the feet at rest or with each step taken. Additionally, a common condition is weakness of the musculature that supports the arch of the foot. With frequent repetitive and high-impact exercises, these misalignments can lead to foot pain, toe cramps, heel discomfort, ankle sprains, and severe foot conditions. The legs, knees, hips, lower back, posture, and spine may also be adversely affected.

Exercising with improper footwear can contribute to or exacerbate these problems. Worn or ill-fitting sneakers do not provide proper foot support, heel cushion, or lateral heel stabilization. Over time, individuals will notice a reduction in the intensity and frequency of their workouts.

If you are serious about exercising and wish to avoid foot problems or are experiencing some of the aforementioned symptoms, you should, at the very least, consider a new pair of sneakers. Make sure they fit comfortably and provide proper support of your foot arch. Many sneakers provide additional support for supination or pronation misalignments. The wear pattern on the soles of your sneakers may indicate a specific problem you may have. It is always a good idea to see a podiatrist if you suspect a foot misalignment or are having persistent foot discomfort. He or she may recommend orthotic inserts that can correct misalignments. A podiatrist can also recommend the best type and brand of sneakers that are right for you.

With the increased popularity of devices that measure the number of steps a person takes daily, more individuals are setting goals of walking ten thousand steps per day to improve their conditioning. Obviously, it makes sense to make every step count as a step in the right direction.

29

We Can Work It Out

Gym Etiquette

Proper gym etiquette is essential for productive and enjoyable workouts. Too often, a lack of basic consideration or rudeness by others can diminish your gym experience. Here are some helpful tips that will help you exemplify yourself as a positive role model at your gym or health club.

Restack And Put Away Your Weights

Always restack your plate weights and return dumbbells to their racks in the correct location. Not everyone uses the same weight as you. Sometimes heavy weights cannot be moved safely by the next person. Weights and dumbbells that are randomly lying around can present a hazard to yourself and others.

Wipe Off Perspiration

Always use a towel to wipe away perspiration and clean an exercise machine after you use it. This is basic hygiene and does not take much effort to do.

Do Not Monopolize Exercise Machines

Avoid spending too much time on one particular exercise machine, cardio equipment, or weight bench. There are others who may be waiting to use the equipment too.

Remember, you would probably not like to slow down or unnecessarily delay your workout for this reason.

Do Not Grunt Or Shout When Lifting

Loud grunting noises and shouting are distracting, rude, and unimpressive to others in the gym.

Avoid Singing Out Loud Or Using A Cell Phone

If you listen to music while working out, try not to sing a particular song out loud. Chances are likely that you probably do not sound very melodic. This can be very annoying and distracting to others. Additionally, leave your cell phone in the locker room.

Avoid Excessive Socialization

While it's OK to meet people and make friends at your gym, try to avoid too much socialization. Not everyone at your gym is looking for social interaction. Excessive socialization can be distracting and disruptive to other members' workouts.

Dress Appropriately

You should make every effort to dress appropriately. Risqué or offensive outfits should not be worn. Men should never work out without wearing a shirt or tank top. Not everyone wants to see too much of you.

30

Homebody

Setting Up a Home Exercise Room

H ome exercise studios are becoming increasingly popular. They allow for the ease of exercising in your own home whenever it is convenient to work out. Traveling to a health club, toting your exercise attire, parking, and unwanted comments by others are no longer problems.

There are several factors to keep in mind when setting up your home exercise room. Too often, people buy the wrong equipment, spend too much money, and end up using the exercise room to hang their laundry.

Measure Your Room Or Space

Take the time to measure the dimensions of your intended exercise room or space. This will allow for proper planning and placement of your exercise equipment.

Research The Exercise Equipment

There are many types of exercise equipment available. Research the equipment to determine if it is what you would like to use and whether it will be effective in achieving your fitness goals.

Measure The Equipment Dimensions

This information is usually included in equipment catalogues and brochures. This information will allow you to properly position your equipment. Don't forget to allow at least three feet around a piece of equipment so that you can use it correctly. Also allow for an area of free space for floor exercises and stretching.

Purchase The Right Equipment For You

Make sure the equipment you purchase is right for you. You may not need an exercise machine with a 1,000-pound capacity if you don't lift anything heavier than 150 pounds. Equipment for single-person use is usually less expensive than commercial-grade equipment found in health clubs.

Set Up Your Exercises Room In Stages

Start with basic equipment, such as free weights, tubes, and stability balls, and gradually add more equipment over time. You will avoid spending too much on equipment that you do not use.

Add TV And Music

A great workout can be done while watching a game or your favorite TV show. Listening to music can keep you relaxed and focused while you exercise.

Dessert

Unique Situations and Special People

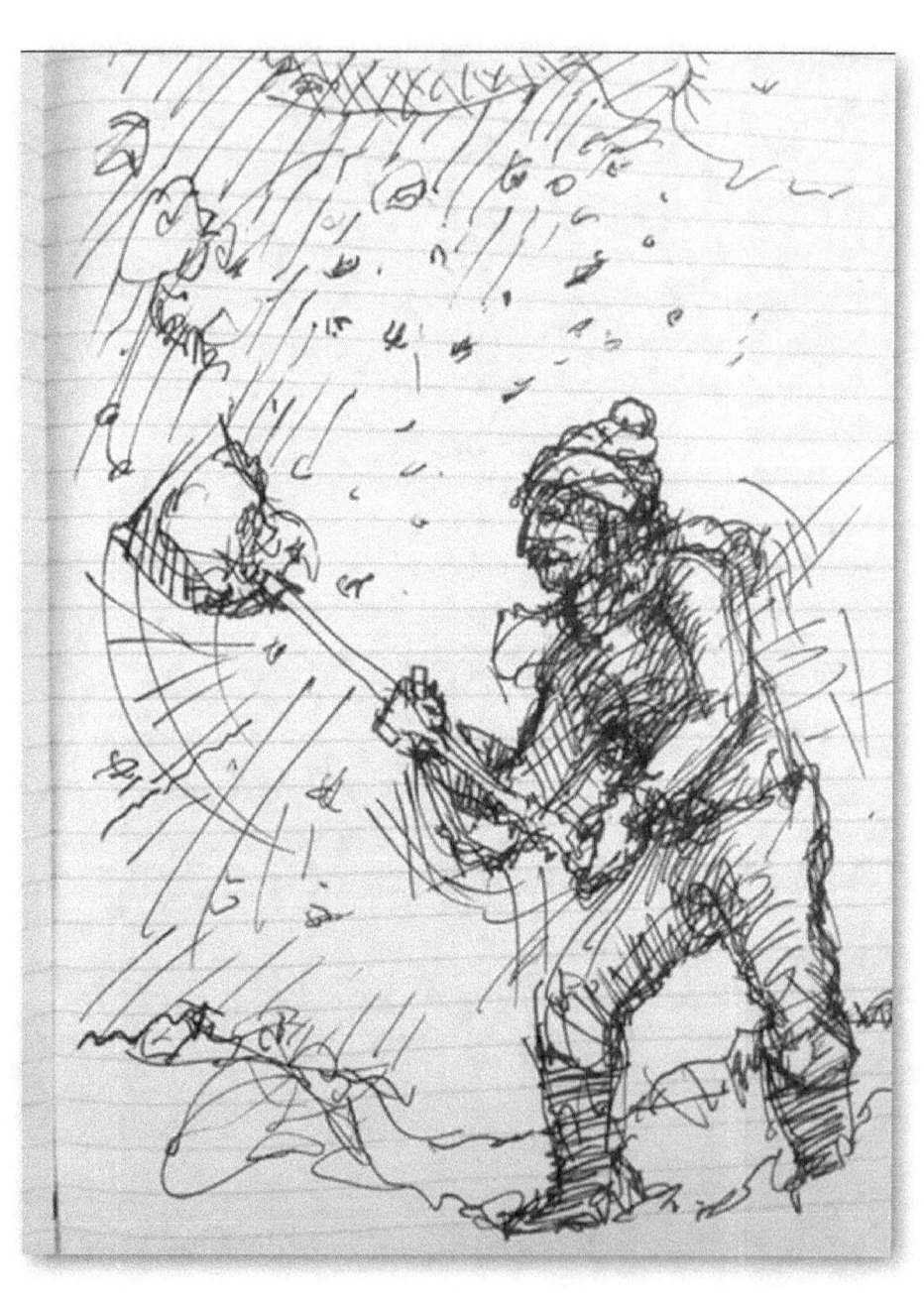

31

Take This Job and Shovel It

Fitness Tips for Snow Removal

Snow removal, especially snow shoveling, can lead to a host of physical discomforts and injury. The sudden strain on your muscles and joints often leads to untimely and costly visits to the doctor. Here are some helpful fitness tips to reduce your chances of sustaining an injury as well as reducing aches and pains.

Use Your Legs
Use your legs to lift a shovel full of snow. Do not rely only on your back muscles. Your legs can provide a great deal of lifting power.

Change Up Your Movements
Change your movement patterns when shoveling snow for an extended period of time. Switch hand positions when holding the shovel. You can also throw the snow in a different direction.

Take A Break
Take a break every fifteen to twenty minutes when shoveling. Also take a break if you feel dizzy or have shortness of breath. If you are unaccustomed to snow shoveling or have not been exercising, break up your snow removal into time periods of no more than thirty to forty minutes.

Drink Plenty Of Water

Drink plenty of water to replenish lost fluids due to the strenuous physical activity associated with snow shoveling. Since it is cold outside, you may not sweat or notice that you are thirsty.

Do Strength-Training Exercises

If you know that snow shoveling is likely this winter, increase your strength-training workouts. Useful exercises are squats, latissimus dorsi pulldowns, seated rows, reverse crunches, and all forms of abdominal movements.

Stretch Before And After You Shovel Snow

As with any demanding physical activity, it is helpful to stretch your muscles both before and after snow shoveling.

32

See How They Run

Fitness for Children

There are some disconcerting trends prevalent in today's society with regard to children's fitness conditioning. Obesity is increasing faster in children under the age of eighteen than in the adult population. Health conditions associated with poor physical conditioning (such as hypertension) that were usually found in adults are now being diagnosed in children. Children's obesity can lead to psychological problems, such as depression and low self-esteem. This may lead to poor performance in school.

There are many reasons for this. Some of them are sedentary lifestyles, large fast-food serving portions, and a lack of emphasis on exercise. Parents and adult relatives are responsible for reversing this trend. While constant direct supervision is not always possible, below are some tips that may help.

Be Aware Of Portion Size Of Your Children's Meals

Try to serve healthy portions of food to your children. Do not force them to eat too much of what you feel is good for them. They will learn to overeat and take this habit with them when they are eating out with their friends.

Teach Healthy Eating Habits

By encouraging healthy eating habits of smaller portions five to six times per day, your children will be less likely to binge or overeat when they are eating out.

Encourage Exercise And Other Physical Activities

Emphasize regular exercise, sports, and outdoor activities with your children. Try to make these activities fun. Do not stress winning or unrealistic results.

Be Supportive And Provide Positive Motivation

Your children will probably be reluctant to exercise. They may also feel that they are wasting time, are inadequate, or cannot do it. Stay positive and provide constant support.

Reward Good Behavior

It is very important to reward your children's efforts to eat right and exercise. This will encourage your children to continue with these behaviors.

Participate In Physical Activities With Your Children

This tip has many commonsense benefits. It provides you with quality time with your children while participating in activities that are beneficial to everyone. Share thirty to sixty minutes of aerobic "play" as often as possible with your children.

Practice What You Preach

Be a role model for the next generation. You will enhance your credibility and establish a healthier lifestyle for yourself as well.

33

It's Mother's Day

Fitness Tips for Moms

t is not easy to raise children and still find the time and energy to exercise. The demands of parenthood are challenging. Nevertheless, it is important to make every effort to take care of yourself both physically and mentally. This will benefit both you and your children. Here are some helpful fitness tips for hardworking moms.

Exercise At Home
Try to set up an area in your home where you can exercise. Simple, inexpensive exercise equipment, such as stability balls and resistance tubes, are very useful. You can supervise your children while simultaneously completing an effective workout. You also do not have to leave your house or leave your children with a babysitter.

Exercise With A Friend
Working out with a friend or relative can be very effective. The company will be mentally and socially stimulating. Exercising with a friend is usually more effective than exercising alone.

Share Child Supervision
Share the supervision of children with a neighbor, friend, relative, or spouse. You could watch your friend's children with your own and allow her to work out. Then she could do the same for you.

Exercise With Your Children

If your children are older, share physical activity with them. It's fun, and you'll get a great workout.

Eat Healthy, Eat Often, And Drink Water

Eat often and drink a lot of water to maintain metabolism. You will feel more energized. Avoid children's snacks that are high in sugar.

Use A Personal Trainer

A personal trainer will help utilize your limited exercise time more efficiently. A personal trainer will also help reduce the stress of trying to figure out what exercises you should do.

34

New Tricks for Old Dogs

Home Exercise Tips for Seniors

Senior citizens are the fastest-growing segment of our national population. Additionally, with advancements in medical treatment, more people are living longer. In order for elderly people to continue to enjoy active and fulfilling lives, it is necessary that they engage in regular exercise.

Use The Stairs As Much As Possible

Go up and down stairs in your home as often as you can. Try to do household chores, such as loading your laundry one item at a time, while repeatedly going up and down the stairs.

Clean And Reorganize Your Kitchen Cabinets And Pantry

Take out all the items in a kitchen cabinet, reorganize them, and then put them back. You will exercise your entire upper body and improve handgrip strength.

Sit On A Stability Ball When You Watch Television

Simply sit as straight up as possible on a stability ball while watching television. You will improve core strength, balance, and posture.

Walk As Much As Possible

Get in the habit of walking outside as much as possible either before or after meals. Use an iPod to listen to your favorite music.

Set Fitness Goals That Are Based On Health, Not Appearance

Become motivated to exercise to improve your health. Do not worry about trying to look young again. Increased fitness will allow you to enjoy your life and participate in more activities with family and friends.

Use A Personal Trainer

A qualified personal trainer who has experience with senior citizens can develop exercise programs that are both safe and effective. He or she can also monitor your progress, keep your workouts interesting, and provide positive motivation.

Take It Easy

Avoid stressful workouts, especially if you exercise alone. Allow yourself plenty of rest and take a break if you feel too tired.

Learn And Do Small Home-Improvement Projects

Learn to do small home-improvement projects and repairs. You will find this both physically and mentally stimulating. You'll also feel a sense of accomplishment and save money.

35

It's Raining Cats and Dogs

Exercise with Your Pets

Many people today own pets. Pets are a source of companionship, joy, and love. They are often considered part of the family. One way to motivate yourself to exercise is to work out or participate in physical activities with your pet. You will find this enjoyable and less of a chore. Since obesity is a common problem with both cats and dogs, your pet will also benefit from the exercise. Left on their own, cats and dogs usually become couch potatoes. Below are some helpful tips.

Run, Jog, Or Walk With Your Dog
This is a great way for you and your pet to engage in aerobic activity. You will find this both challenging and enjoyable. Make sure both you and your pet have enough water to drink and take it easy if either one of you feels exhausted.

Go Up And Down The Stairs With Your Cat
Cats, by nature, are more independent and will not always follow you when participating in activities. However, you can use some catnip or a new cat toy to entice your cat to walk up a flight of stairs. When you both reach the top, you can throw the catnip or toy down the stairs. Your cat will most likely follow you back down. Repeat this routine for a great workout.

Chase Your Pet Around Your House Or Apartment

It is a fun idea to chase your pet playfully around your house or apartment. You can also have your pet chase you. Catnip, food, toys, and the expectation of a reward can help with motivation. The quick lateral movements usually associated with chasing games will burn calories and improve your balance.

Play Catch With Your Pet

Use a ball, your pet's favorite toy, or any object to play catch with your pet. This usually works best with dogs; however, cats may go after a bag of catnip. When you are outside with your dog, use a Frisbee as a fun alternative.

36

Taking Care of Business

Exercise and Fitness at the Office

Many of us spend the majority of our time at work. Frequently, our careers demand priority attention, and we don't always have the time to work out. Below are some helpful suggestions to stay in shape during the workday.

Move Around And Change Your Position
If you find yourself at a desk sitting in the same position, try to get up and move around every fifteen to twenty minutes. You should change up any repetitive motions, such as doing routine tasks, in a different order and, if possible, take a different route when moving from one office room to another.

Use The Stairs
If you have to go up one or two floors, use the stairs instead of an escalator or an elevator. Use the stairs when leaving work or going out.

Stretch
Stretch out your large muscles periodically during the day. This only takes a few minutes but will relieve muscle strain and soreness.

Tighten Up Your Abs

While you are sitting at a desk or standing up, do several sets of isometric abdominal contractions. You should do one to three sets of six to fifteen contractions. Hold each contraction for a minimum of five seconds.

Sit Up Straight

Always remind yourself to sit up straight in your chair, especially when using a computer for an extended period of time.

Go Out For Lunch Or Bring Your Own; Avoid Food Delivery

Going out for lunch allows you time to walk. The time walking will cut down on your eating time, and hopefully you'll consume less. If you bring a healthy lunch from home, walk around for the balance of your lunch break. Try to avoid ordering in large lunches or working through your lunch break.

Take Walking Breaks

If possible, try to take one or two fifteen-minute breaks and walk around, preferably out of your office. If your office has an accessible rooftop, use the stairwell and go up for some fresh air.

37

Roam around the World

Fitness Tips for Travel

Travel, whether it is for business or pleasure, is often a time when many people cannot or will not engage in physical activity. However, there are benefits to exercising while you are away. Increased energy and mental alertness as well as reduced travel fatigue are just a few. Below are some simple tips to help you in your travels.

Stretch In Your Seat

On long flights, it is good idea to periodically stretch. This will help reduce muscle stiffness and improve circulation. Holding a stretch for twenty or thirty seconds is the best method.

Drink Water And Avoid Alcohol

Stay hydrated throughout your journey. Drinking water will keep your metabolism up and help you avoid fatigue. Drinking alcohol will add empty calories to your diet and result in undesirable weight gain.

Bring Energy Bars On Long Flights

Airplane food is usually high in carbohydrates. Food is also served infrequently, especially in coach class. Bring a supply of healthy snacks with you. This is helpful to avoid long periods between meals.

Don't Use The People Mover

Walking and movement in general are smart and healthy activities after a long flight. They restore circulation, boost metabolism, and burn calories.

Pack A Set Of Exercise Tubes

Exercise tubes are lightweight, easy to use, and provide a wide variety of resistance exercises. They can be used in your hotel room for brief but effective workouts.

38

Running after a Runny Nose

Exercise Tips after a Cold or the Flu

During the winter months, many healthy people will experience colds, the flu, nasal congestion, sinus inflammation, and flu-like symptoms. Resuming exercise before there is a complete recovery from illness can lead to a relapse and poor results. Here are some commonsense tips for resuming workouts after being sick.

Don't Rush It
Make sure you feel completely better before you return to your exercise routines. In some cases, especially when you have been sick for over a week, allow a few days of good health to pass before starting up again.

Don't Push It
Reduce the intensity level and duration of your first few workouts after recovering from an illness. Do not attempt to make up for lost time by overdoing it.

Go Easy With Cardiovascular Workouts
Avoid vigorous cardiovascular workouts immediately after recovering from a cold, the flu, or another respiratory condition. Increased breathing intensity may irritate bronchial and nasal tissues, resulting in a return of respiratory inflammation.

Wait Until You Are Finished With Medications

Do not restart your exercise workouts until you have finished any prescription medicine or over-the-counter medications. Consult with your doctor if necessary.

Stay Inside If The Weather Is Cold

In cold climates, avoid outdoor cardiovascular exercise. The increased stress on your body will weaken your immune system and lead to a relapse.

Listen To Your Body

Be acutely aware of your physical condition and symptoms. If you are unusually tired, sense a return of any type of symptom, or just don't feel "right," back off from your workouts and rest.

Don't Worry

Don't worry that you have become out of shape because you've done nothing while you were sick. As your health improves, so will your level of conditioning. After a complete recovery, your workouts will also return to your previous level of performance.

39

Eat, Drink, and Don't Be Heavy

Fitness Tips for the Holiday Season

Increase Your Workout Intensity Before Thanksgiving

During the entire month of November, try to increase the length, frequency, and intensity of your workouts. After Thanksgiving, you may have more family, social, and shopping commitments, which may infringe on your workout time.

Cut Back On Calories Before The Holidays

Reduce your overall caloric intake about a month before Thanksgiving. This will allow more leeway to treat yourself and enjoy holiday meals.

Do Quick Workouts

During the holiday season, when you have less time to exercise, do quick workouts. They will keep you in shape and maintain your metabolism. Fifteen to twenty minutes is better than not working out at all.

Park Far Away From The Shopping-Mall Entrance

You can get an aerobic workout briskly walking the extra distance and actually save time looking for a parking spot.

Use Stairs Instead Of The Escalator

This is a quick way to burn a few more calories when you're shopping.

Have A Light Snack Before A Holiday Party

Try to eat a light, healthy snack and drink plenty of water before you attend a holiday or office party. You will be less likely to binge or overeat, and you'll keep your metabolism up for greater caloric expenditure.

Eat A Healthy Breakfast

Take your time to eat a full, healthy breakfast. This is always a good idea; however, during the holidays, when you may be under greater stress or may be more tempted to overeat, a good breakfast will help you avoid overindulgence and give you the energy to keep shopping.

Ease Up On Alcohol Consumption

Alcohol contains seven calories per gram. Try to avoid drinking too much of it to prevent excessive caloric intake. If you plan to drive, it is imperative that you avoid it altogether.

40

You Say You Want a Resolution

New Fitness Tips for the New Year

The beginning of a new year is traditionally a time when people decide to make some changes in their physical appearance and fitness conditioning. Here are some helpful tips to get you started and maintain your workouts through the year.

Schedule Your Workouts

It is important to keep your workouts regular. Time management is often a problem, especially at the beginning of an exercise program. Workouts should be scheduled as appointments, and unless you are ill, you should make every effort to keep them.

Set Realistic Goals

Try to keep your short, intermediate, and long-term goals realistic. Do not become obsessed with too-rapid weight loss or excessive muscle gain. Keeping your fitness goals realistic will keep you motivated and prevent depression from a perceived failure to achieve the results you expect.

Get A Checkup From Your Doctor

If you have not had a physical for over a year, it is a good idea to get a checkup from your doctor before you begin to exercise regularly. This is also true for individuals who have been working out for an extended period of time.

Emphasize The Health Benefits Of Exercise

Improved personal health should be the most important long-term goal that everyone should have. Always keep in mind that the main reason you are working out is to stay healthy.

Try Something New

There are many different types of workouts, exercise classes, training methods, and fitness products available to use or participate in. Try something that you have only thought about but have never actually done.

Use A Personal Trainer

To achieve maximum results, avoid injury, save time, and stay motivated, use the services of a personal fitness professional.

41

Buns in the Oven

Fitness Tips for Pregnancy

Numerous studies have indicated that mild to moderate exercise is of great benefit to pregnant women. Exercise during pregnancy helps maintain muscle strength, reduce excessive weight gain, and maintain optimal levels of physical and mental health. Usually, women can continue their normal exercise during the first trimester without much difficulty. During the second and third trimesters, exercise intensity, duration, and frequency should be reduced, and certain guidelines listed below should be followed. While pregnant, it is always important to stay properly hydrated, eat a small snack before exercising to avoid hypoglycemia, and stop exercising if any dizziness, unusual physical changes, sickness, or other problems occur. Of course, during the entire term of pregnancy, it is necessary to discuss exercise plans and goals with a physician.

Extend Warm-Up And Cooldown Sessions
Take extra time to warm up and cool down. This will allow the body to maintain a more stable temperature, heart rate, and blood pressure.

Avoid Exercise When The Temperature Is High
Body temperature should not exceed one hundred degrees Fahrenheit during pregnancy. Temperature should be checked immediately after exercise. Avoid exercising in hot weather or humidity. This will help keep the body at a safe temperature.

Reduce Range Of Motion And Excessive Stretching

With the release of the hormone relaxin during pregnancy, joints become looser, thus increasing the risk of injury. Therefore, a pregnant woman should limit her range of motion, especially while performing resistance exercises.

Avoid Exercise In The Supine Position

Exercise in the supine position (face up or on your back) should be performed with caution during the first trimester and should be avoided during the second and third trimesters. This prevents excessive pressure on the fetus and on the mother's spine.

Wear Supportive Shoes

Wearing good, supportive shoes while pregnant will help reduce foot problems and leg fatigue.

Avoid Excessive Impact Activities

Activities such as running, jogging, and step classes should be avoided. Alternative forms of aerobic exercise, such as swimming and bicycling, are preferable and safer.

42

All Stuffed Up

Exercise Tips for the Allergy Season

The late winter, spring, and early summer are considered the allergy season in large parts of the country. Many people suffer from allergies that result in a host of symptoms that can be uncomfortable and, at times, debilitating. Allergic reactions and allergy medicine can often affect your exercise performance.

Exercise Indoors

If possible, do your workouts indoors at a gym or in your home. A controlled, filtered environment will have a lower allergen concentration than the outside.

Avoid Intense Aerobic Activity

If you are suffering from allergy symptoms, avoid intense aerobic activity. You may find it difficult to breathe at intense levels of exertion. Heavy respiration could worsen your allergic reactions.

Check With Your Physician Regarding Medications

If you take medication for a specific allergy condition, check with your physician before you exercise. There may be side effects from your medication that could affect your performance. Also, intense exercise may exacerbate the harmful side effects of certain anti-allergy medications.

Take Extra Time To Stretch

Your muscles may feel stiff or sore as a result of your body's histamine response to some types of allergens. Take extra time to gently stretch your muscles before, during, and after your workouts.

Reduce Your Resistance Level

It is a good idea to back off on your resistance level or the weight you lift if you are suffering from allergies or are taking medication. Fatigue, slower reaction times, and lethargy are common symptoms of both allergies and allergy medications. You simply may not be able to focus and keep up a sustained intensity during your workouts. Take it easy until your symptoms improve and you feel better.

Leftovers

Live a Healthy and Happy Lifestyle

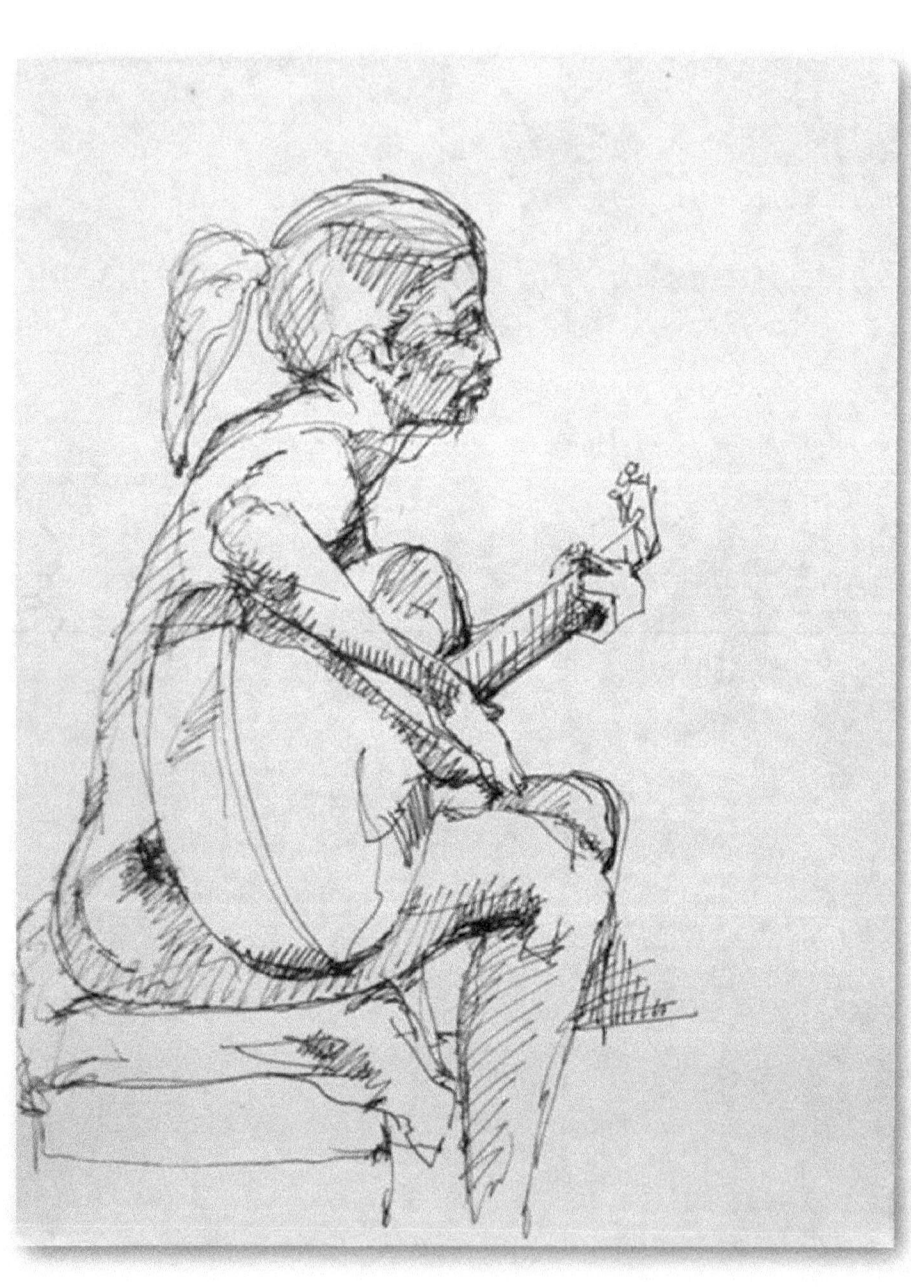

43

Young at Heart

Rediscover Your Inner Child

All people age. It's a fact of life. Often, we look back on our youth with fond memories and wish we could be like kids again. At our current level of technology, we are not yet able to travel back in time to when we were children. However, if we embrace a positive attitude and adopt the following simple suggestions, it is possible to feel young again.

Play With Your Friends

When we were children, we always enjoyed playtime with our friends. Even though we are older, it is still fun to get together with friends and play. The playtime activities may change, but it is still fun to meet a friend, take a walk, or do something that you both enjoy.

Play With Your Toys

Children love to have toys. However, it is also fun, even as adults, to play with toys—they just may cost more. Some fun toys that we can still enjoy are hula hoops, roller skates, and trampolines. These toys provide excellent exercise alternatives.

Play With Your Children

Playing with your children provides so many benefits. You are active, spending quality time with your children, and, once again, enjoying the simple pleasure of playtime.

Go Dancing

Dancing is an excellent activity for burning calories. When we were younger, especially as teenagers and young adults, we enjoyed a lot of social enjoyment when we went out dancing. Dancing brings us together with those we love. We can again enjoy our favorite music and relive the fun we had in our youth.

44

Don't Worry; Be Happy

Accept Reality and Set Realistic Goals

There is one reality common for everybody: we are all getting older. Too often, people deny this inevitable process, and, for some, depression can result from refusing to accept this inescapable fact. People often let themselves go, which can result in excessive weight gain, health problems, and poor quality of life. Below are some simple guidelines that will hopefully lead to a happier and healthier life at any age.

Be Happy With Your Age

Accept your age and be comfortable with it. There are unique benefits and enjoyment at all ages. As one grows older, the wisdom obtained from life experiences can be shared with those younger than you. This will enrich their lives and yours as well.

Don't Compete With Your Past

Do not constantly compare your physical appearance and ability to when you were younger. Time waits for no one, and physiological changes are inevitable. Instead, concentrate on being the best you can be at your current age.

Don'T Compare Yourself To Models And Celebrities

Most models and celebrities live a different life than the average person. They usually can devote more time to long workouts, beauty treatments, and cosmetic surgery.

When they are photographed, the photos are usually taken professionally and are enhanced with extensive digital editing.

Learn From Your Mistakes

One of the benefits of aging is that you have hopefully learned from your past mistakes and experiences. You can apply this knowledge to manage your time better. Your exercise workouts will be more effective and efficient.

Avoid Injury

Accept and know your physical limitations and do not be in denial. This mind-set will help you to avoid injury. Recovery from injury becomes more problematic as one gets older.

45

If You're a Couch Potato, Then Be a Fritter Instead

TV Calories

Watching television is a common activity for people of all ages. While the cultural benefits of television are debatable, one thing is certain: watching television leads to a more sedentary lifestyle. The popular expression "couch potato" describes a person who sits and watches television. This can lead to low metabolism, low caloric expenditure, and greater weight gain.

Recent observations indicate that people who fidget may burn almost five hundred additional calories per day than someone who does not. Therefore, if you can increase your physical activity or move around while watching television, you could burn more calories and avoid weight gain. Below are some useful suggestions.

Clean Your House Or Apartment

While watching television, if you can, clean your house or apartment. Push a vacuum around, dust, and straighten out your living room or den. This will burn calories, and you gain the benefit of a cleaner home.

Install A Television In The Kitchen Or Garage

If you install a television in the kitchen or garage, you can watch television while doing other tasks. You can complete chores, burn calories, and watch your favorite program all at the same time.

Be The Host

Invite family and friends over to watch your favorite television programs or sporting events. You will probably have to get up more often to be hospitable. Again, you will burn more calories and increase your popularity.

Get Up During Commercials

Instead of channel surfing during commercials, get up and move around.

Do Not Eat And Watch Television

This is often difficult to avoid. You should try not to eat large meals while watching television and limit your consumption to light snacks.

46

An Affair to Remember

Event Motivation

One of the biggest challenges people face when they engage in regular exercise is staying motivated. Results often come more slowly than hoped for, and people tend to give up on exercise. For others, the perceived monotony of their workouts causes them to slack off and exercise with less intensity. Also, due to lack of motivation, people have a hard time getting started with an exercise program and avoid physical activity altogether.

Everyone goes through periods of time when their motivation to exercise varies. Besides the previously stated examples of decreased motivation, there are times when motivation is higher. These increased levels of motivation are commonly associated with specific times or upcoming special events.

If a person is going to participate in a wedding, he or she will become more motivated to lose weight in order to fit into a favorite outfit or look good in the wedding pictures. This is particularly true if it is that person's own wedding or that of a family member.

The start of a new year and the beginning of summer are examples of specific times when people generally have increased motivation to exercise and lose weight. New Year's resolutions or the desire to look better in a bathing suit usually lead to an increase in health club memberships and a more focused effort to eat healthier.

If you make a list of events for each season of the year, you can stay motivated and avoid frequent periods of inactivity. Besides traditional New Year's resolutions, weddings, class reunions, office parties, birthdays, and family gatherings, below are some examples of seasonal events that can be used for motivation.

Spring

- Lose weight gained in the winter.
- Increase physical conditioning for outdoor activities.

Summer

- Get in shape for summer clothing.
- Exercise to increase physical activities, especially with children.

Autumn

- Exercise to improve sport-specific performance.
- Get back in shape after a summer vacation.

Winter

- Prevent weight gain from overeating during the holidays.
- Get in better shape for vacations in the tropics.

47

Hey, You Can Hide Your Blubber Away

Fashion Tips to Look Slimmer

Proper diet and exercise are the cornerstones of a healthy lifestyle. However, weight loss and weight management are often difficult for most people to achieve quickly. Too often, we stare in the mirror and are not happy with the pace of desired results. Sometimes, it is helpful to dress to look thinner. While this obviously does not lead directly to weight loss, it can boost self-confidence and self-esteem. These benefits can help sustain motivation and eventually aid in actual weight loss. Here are some tips that can help you look slimmer.

Choose The Right Clothes

select clothing that accentuates your best features. Avoid clothing that draws attention to problem areas. For instance, if you are trying to lose weight in your legs, wear dark-colored pants and avoid brightly colored garments.

Proper Fit

Clothing that fits properly will help you looks slimmer. When it comes to size selection, keep in mind that there are size variations between different styles and manufacturers. Not all size-twelve clothing has the same specifications. Do not try to fit into a smaller size just for the sake of a number.

Avoid Tight Or Clingy Garments

Certain materials such as wool and cotton usually do not fit tightly and allow room for easy movement. Garments made from these fabrics will not conform tightly to your figure. Fabrics such as nylon or spandex will cling to your body tighter and show every bulge. "Stretch" garments will also cling tightly to your figure.

48

Nip and Tuck

Thoughts on Cosmetic Surgery

Cosmetic surgery has become more common in recent times. People are electing to have surgical procedures to correct minor physical imperfections or improve their appearances. Others elect to have cosmetic surgery to eliminate undesirable physical conditions that have developed over time. For some, cosmetic surgery is necessary to restore damaged or diseased body parts.

Surgery, whether it is a minor procedure or a major operation, always has an element of risk. An individual who is considering any type of cosmetic surgery should have a clear understanding of these risks. Make sure your surgeon explains the particular risks of your surgery and answers all your questions. It is also important to remember that even with simple procedures, it is imperative that you choose an experienced, well-qualified surgeon. Thoroughly check your surgeon's credentials and background. Be wary of a surgeon or a plastic-surgery practice that offer discounts or "specials" for cosmetic surgery.

Cosmetic surgery should not be a shortcut for physical improvement. It should be considered only if regular exercise and proper diet have not yielded the results you want. These results should always be realistic. An obsessive desire for perfection is not a good reason to have cosmetic surgery. If you honestly feel you're doing the best you can to stay healthy, then cosmetic surgery may be considered for additional personal enhancement.

49

Genes That Fit

How Genetics Can Affect Your Fitness

In the last few years, the human genome largely has been mapped out. This remarkable achievement will lead to a better understanding and treatment of many diseases that have, up to now, eluded a cure. It also appears that research has begun to establish a correlation between an individual's genes and fitness level.

Many research studies using families have found significant similarities in body composition, cholesterol levels, and blood pressure. A thirty-year study on exercise response involving two hundred families, conducted by Dr. Claude Bouchard of the Pennington Biomedical Research Center at Louisiana State University, concluded that there was three times greater variance in maximal oxygen uptake levels between families than within families. Clearly, genetics is a factor in these results.

It should be no surprise to many of us that fitness levels and appearance vary greatly in individuals who engage in similar workouts. Some people develop significant increases in muscle mass no matter what type of resistance training they perform, while others hardly change in appearance despite intense workouts.

This information may be discouraging to some. However, a more positive outlook is that we use these findings as a rationale for setting realistic fitness goals. We should not be overly obsessed with obtaining levels of muscle bulk, weight loss, or physical appearance that are biologically impossible to achieve. We should concentrate on improving our health, maximizing our own unique physical potential, and playing the game of life as best as we can with the hand that was dealt to us.

50

Now It's Time to Say Good Night

Helpful Tips for Sleep

A restful night's sleep is essential for good physical and mental health. Everyone, at some time, experiences sleep disruption, sleep deprivation, or insomnia. However, in many instances these problems develop into a chronic pattern. These individuals are fatigued, cannot exercise properly, and suffer decreased results and performance. Without help, medical problems can arise. Below are some tips for getting a good night's sleep.

Go To Sleep And Wake Up At The Same Time

Try to keep regular hours. Wake up at the same time every day, whether you have to get up for work or not. In the evening, go to bed at the same time. Don't stay up late.

Do Not Oversleep To Make Up For Lost Sleep

If you did not get enough sleep on a particular night, do not oversleep the next morning to make up for it. You will have trouble falling asleep later that night.

Avoid Exercise At Least One Hour Before Bedtime

Try not to exercise too late in the evening. End your workouts at least one hour before your bedtime. Exercise increases metabolism, and you may find it difficult to relax.

Avoid Alcohol, Caffeine, And Stimulants

Reduce your consumption of alcohol, caffeine, and stimulants, especially after midafternoon. Try to eliminate an alcoholic nightcap before bedtime. Alcohol decreases REM sleep, which is the deep, restful, dream sleep your brain and body need.

Avoid Watching The Nightly News

Avoid watching the nightly news broadcast prior to going to sleep. Too often, the negative images and stories can be upsetting and prevent you from falling asleep. Instead, read a relaxing book or listen to soothing music.

Avoid Serious Discussions

If possible, try to avoid discussing important matters with your spouse, roommate, or significant other just before bedtime. Explain your sleep problem and agree to set aside a more convenient time to talk.

Write Down The Next Day's Business And Necessary Tasks

Prior to bedtime, write down any important things that need to be done for the next day. This will help you avoid thinking about them as you try to fall asleep.

Seek Professional Help

Many new sleep-disorder therapies are available today. Sleep centers can analyze and diagnose your particular sleep problem and provide a cure. Ask your physician for specific information on available sleep-therapy options.

About the Author

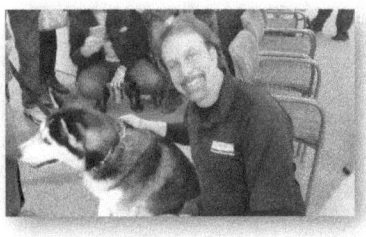

V

ince Lambri's involvement with health and fitness began when he graduated from Stony Brook University. At that time, he embarked on a career as a health-care professional. In order to keep himself in shape and relieve the stress of career responsibilities, he attempted to work out at various fitness centers and health clubs. However, he often found that he stagnated in his workout routines. Then he began to exercise regularly with a certified personal trainer. His trainer's expertise and motivation changed his exercise experience entirely. He soon looked forward to working out and enjoyed exercising. Most importantly, he saw real changes in his physique and felt healthier than ever. In short, he saw results. Finally, he broke through his exercise and fitness plateaus—something Vince had not been able to achieve on his own.

Vince found himself increasingly interested in the science of resistance training, nutrition, weight training, and exercising. He was surprised to learn that there is a tremendous amount of information concerning exercise and physical fitness. He earnestly studied the science of exercise and fitness and became a certified personal trainer with the National Academy of Sports Medicine. Expanding on his fitness and nutritional knowledge, Vince furthered his studies and education by achieving an MBA in health-care management.

For the past twenty-two years, Vince has been personally training many different types of people in his private exercise studio, at individuals' homes, and at health clubs throughout New York, New Jersey, and Connecticut. He was the owner of two Curves for Women franchises in Connecticut and a former executive director at Healthrax

Fitness and Wellness. Currently, Vince is an instructor at Branford Hall Career Institute and at the World Instructor Training Schools. He is also a member of the elite personal training staff at Snap Fitness in Avon, Connecticut, and a Certified Coach with The Body Lab in Newington, Connecticut.

Vince's personal fitness philosophy is quite simple: "Everybody can improve their health, appearance, and lifestyle regardless of their age, athletic ability, or medical history. Making it happen is the real challenge and reward of being a fitness professional."